GLUCOSE REFORMISM:

A guide on what to eat, improve and balance your body glucose

BY: Bettye B. Atlas

CHAPTER 1

GLUCOSE

Your body uses this particular sort of sugar, which it obtains from the food you consume, as fuel. It is referred to as blood glucose or blood sugar when it passes through your bloodstream to reach your cells. When

your blood sugar levels are under control, they frequently go unnoticed. However, they can have an impact on how your body functions on a daily basis when they grow or dip excessively. So, what exactly is glucose?

It is a monosaccharide, which is a form of carbohydrate that is the most basic and means "one sugar."

Galactose, ribose, and fructose are examples of additional monosaccharides. The body gradually transforms food glucose and other carbohydrates into

blood glucose in this form. Among the body's main fuel sources, along with fat and protein, is glucose. The term "sugar" refers to a wide variety of caloric sweeteners in various sorts and forms. Table sugar is the most widely used kind of sugar. According to science, table sugar is sucrose, a disaccharide made up of an equal mixture of fructose and glucose, two monosaccharides.

Monosaccharides, which are solitary sugar molecules, are frequently referred to as "simple" sugars. We eat fructose, galactose, and glucose as our three primary monosaccharides. The three types of disaccharides (two connected sugar units) that are most crucial for human nutrition are lactose, maltose, and sucrose, which combine in a variety of combinations. The link between all of these is glucose.

What is the source of glucose?

The most prevalent monosaccharide in nature is glucose. It is produced by photosynthesis in plants. Chains of linked glucose are stored by some plants. Starch is the name for these chains. Foods that frequently contain starch include corn, potatoes, rice, and wheat. From these entire food sources, starch is professionally separated to create dextrose, glucose, maltodextrins, polyols, and high fructose corn syrup, which are then used as ingredients in the creation of a variety of foods, drinks, dressings, and sauces.

Some foods naturally include glucose monosaccharides, however not as part of the starch component. Honey and dried fruits including dates, apricots, raisins, currants, cranberries, prunes, and figs are the two sources of

glucose monosaccharides that are found in the highest concentration in whole foods.

Is glucose added or natural sugar?

Depending on where it comes from, the sugar we eat is either referred to as natural sugar or added sugar. If glucose is taken straight from whole foods like apricots and dates, it is regarded as a natural sugar. When consumed from packaged foods and beverages to which it has been added during manufacture, glucose is regarded as an added sugar. Sadly, just approximately one in ten persons in America consumes the recommended daily amounts of fruits and vegetables, while six out of ten consume more added sugars than is healthy.

How is glucose broken down?

Technically, glucose does not need to be digested. Instead, it enters the bloodstream through the small intestine and is immediately absorbed, where it can either be converted to energy or eventually stored as glycogen in the liver and muscle. We obtain glucose via foods and drinks that contain lactose, sucrose, and starch as well as straight from foods like honey. When we consume foods high in starch, our saliva must first convert the starch to maltose (pairs of linked glucose units). The individual glucose units in maltose are then further broken down, releasing them for absorption. When we consume lactose and sucrose, glucose is digested similarly to how maltose is digested before being absorbed after being split from its monosaccharide companion. (Fructose is found in sucrose and galactose in lactose). Disaccharide and starch digestion take longer

than glucose absorption, which causes less of a blood sugar spike than taking in glucose immediately.

Can the body produce glucose?

Glucose is necessary for our bodies to function. Given that our brain consumes roughly 60% of the glucose that our bodies consume, it is very important for this organ. But glucose doesn't always have to come from food and drink right away. The body produces its own glucose to make sure we always have plenty. By dissolving glycogen to release the glucose it contains, this can be accomplished. Between meals or during times of vigorous exercise, glycogen is broken down. The process of gluconeogenesis, which is mostly carried out by the liver, allows the body to create glucose from non-carbohydrate sources. When glucose production is too

low or nonexistent and glycogen stores are depleted, as happens during extended fasting or starvation, gluconeogenesis takes place.

How is glucose processed by the body?

Ideally, your body uses glucose several times each day.

When you eat, it gets to work right away breaking down glucose and other carbohydrates. The pancreas then aids enzymes as they start to break them down.

Your body's ability to process glucose depends on the production of hormones like insulin by the pancreas.

Your body instructs the pancreas to release insulin after eating to control the growing blood sugar level. Then, glucose is used for energy by muscle, fat, and other cells, or it is stored as fat for later use.

When the pancreas doesn't generate insulin as it should, diabetes may result. To process and control glucose in the body in this situation, you might need outside assistance (insulin injections).

According to a 2018 analysis, insulin resistance may potentially lead to diabetes. When this happens, too much sugar remains in the bloodstream because the body's cells are unable to detect insulin.

your body doesn't react to insulin as it should, glucose can't get into your cells to be used as energy. Your body reacts by directing your cells to produce ketones, which happens at night and while you're fasting or dieting.

Your insulin levels may eventually drop if you have insulin resistance, according to the American Diabetes Association (ADA).

Additionally, your body may expel fat from fat cells. The liver also continues to release more ketones, which causes your blood pH to become acidic.

According to the ADA, the development of ketones and change in blood pH may become problematic when your body is unable to utilize glucose as it should. Ketoacidosis is the name for this condition. It is a serious, potentially fatal consequence of diabetes that needs prompt medical attention.

CHAPTER 2

How is blood glucose measured?

According to the ADA, it's critical for diabetics to check their blood glucose levels. How frequently and when blood sugar levels are checked should depend on the needs and objectives of each person with diabetes.

Consult your doctor about how often and when to check your blood sugar levels to remain on top of things. Your doctor might advise evaluating the levels:

• Before and following meals

• prior to and following exercise;

• during prolonged or vigorous exercise

Before going to bed, when beginning a new drug regimen or insulin schedule, when beginning a new work schedule, and when crossing time zones.

Setting glucose level objectives requires discussion with your doctor because they depend on your condition as well as other variables including age and medical history.

One of the most popular ways for people with diabetes to test their blood glucose at home is with a straightforward blood test, according to the National Institute of Diabetes and Digestive and Kidney Diseases.

How to using a blood glucose meter:

1. Prick the side of your fingertip with a tiny lancet needle to produce a drop of blood.

2. Squeeze some blood onto a test strip.

3. Insert the strip into the device.

4. The meter displays the amount of glucose that is now in your blood.

Checking glucose levels continuously

You might want to think about asking your doctor about utilizing a continuous glucose monitoring (CGM) system when managing your diabetes. Your glucose is automatically monitored by the device around-the-clock.

It transmits readings to a monitor using a small sensor that is inserted just beneath the skin, typically on the stomach or arm. Your blood glucose levels are continuously monitored by a CGM, which also notifies you when it rises or falls abnormally. The gadget has several advantages, including:

 requires fewer finger pricks;

 improves glucose management

• results in fewer crises

The majority of CGM users have type 1 diabetes. However, specialists are investigating how it might benefit others, including individuals with type 2 diabetes.

What are the anticipated glucose levels?

To maintain your body functioning at its best, it's critical to keep your blood glucose levels close to the expected range. Diabetes sufferers would need to exercise considerably greater caution.

For those without diabetes, a blood glucose level of fewer than 100 mg/dL on an empty stomach is recommended by a 2021 review.

Two hours after a meal, it ought to be less than 140 mg/dL. The target glucose levels for diabetics are variable because, as was already said, they are tailored to each person's unique circumstances. Together with you, your doctor will develop your treatment objectives.

Several causes for an increase in blood sugar levels are offered by the Centers for Disease Control and Prevention (CDC).

Some of these triggers are:

• Sunburn: Stress brought on by a sunburn may raise blood glucose levels.

• Coffee: Even a black cup of coffee can make you more susceptible to caffeine's effects on blood sugar.

• Missing breakfast may cause your blood sugar levels to rise after lunch and dinner.

• Time of day: Your body has a harder time controlling glucose as the day goes on. The dawn phenomenon, or early morning hormonal surge, may result in a blood sugar increase.

• Medications: Some medicines and nasal sprays may cause your liver to produce more glucose or stop the production of insulin.

• Stress: Excessive strain and concern may raise blood sugar levels.

These are merely some potential triggers. Activity and illness are two more. If you believe your blood sugar is not being properly regulated, try asking your doctor for advice.

Chapter 3

How to react if your glucose level is too high or low

Hypoglycemia, or too low a blood sugar level, and hyperglycemia, or too high a blood sugar level, are both medical terms.

Hypoglycemia

When a glucose level falls below 70 mg/dL, it is too low. Hypoglycemia is another name for this syndrome, which has the potential to be quite serious.

When your blood sugar drops, there are symptoms to look out for. These include: tremors, exhaustion, bewilderment, anxiousness, and sweating.

Taking more of some diabetes drugs than is recommended for you can lead to hypoglycemia. It might also occur if you consume less calories than you need each day or workout longer or harder than usual. It can occasionally happen to people without diabetes as well.

Consuming food or juice can help raise blood glucose levels. Your doctor might work with you to create a strategy, which might include keeping glucose tablets on hand, for when your blood sugar levels are too low (or high).

Hypoglycemia may be fatal if untreated. When that happens, you might require emergency care.

Hyperglycemia

The term hyperglycemia is another name for high blood sugar. This could occur if your body doesn't produce enough insulin or uses it improperly.

The ADA defines blood glucose levels above 130 mg/dL before a meal as being above goal. The ADA now recommends a goal range of 180 mg/dL one to two hours after eating. You should discuss your personal target ranges with your doctor.

The following are some signs of hyperglycemia to watch out for:

- elevated glucose levels in the urine

- urinating frequently

- heightened thirst

Numerous factors determine the normal blood glucose range for you. The best way to be sure you're inside a healthy range is to speak with your doctor.

Hyperglycemia might have additional causes besides uncontrolled diabetes. For instance, stress and anxiety may result in irregular diabetes management. Increased blood glucose levels may result from this.

Diet and exercise may also aid in keeping your blood sugar levels within the desired range. However, there are several circumstances where exercise is inappropriate

and insulin may be required. The best way to control your blood sugar should be discussed with your doctor.

What occurs if the glucose level is not controlled?

Poor glucose management over time has a harmful impact on your health. When your blood sugar levels are consistently high, you could start to notice the following:

- Hands and feet that are numb and tingly

- Heart conditions

- coma

  severe dehydration

joint and extremities pain

blindness

skin infections

Hyperglycemic hyperosmolar syndrome and diabetic ketoacidosis are two further serious side effects. Both ailments are connected to diabetes.

When it falls too low, you can encounter:

Loss of consciousness

Coma

death

• Discuss your symptoms with your healthcare provider if you think you could have diabetes.

GLUCOSE FUNCTION

Glycolysis, gluconeogenesis, glycogenolysis, and glycogenesis are only a few of the mechanisms that go into glucose metabolism. A process called glycolysis occurs in the liver and involves a number of enzymes that promote glucose catabolism in cells. The enzyme

glucokinase in particular enables the liver to sense changes in serum glucose levels and use glucose when they occur, such as after eating. The process of gluconeogenesis occurs when there is no glucose consumption, such as when a person is fasting and sleeping.

• Gluconeogenesis is the process by which glucose is produced in the mitochondria of liver cells using non-carbohydrate components. Additionally, the pancreas releases glucagon during fasting times, which triggers the glycogenolysis process. Glycogen, which is glucose that has been stored, is converted into glucose during glycogenolysis.

Glycogen is created through the process known as glycogenesis, which takes place when the liver has an excess of carbohydrates.

• The circadian cycle regulates glucose tolerance. Humans often reach their maximum glucose tolerance in the morning. The oral glucose tolerance trough occurs in the afternoon and evening. Due to the fact that glycogen storage components peak in the evening and pancreatic beta-cells are most responsive in the morning, this dip probably occurs. The afternoon is when adipose tissue is most responsive to insulin. The cycle of glucose metabolism is made up of the several times when fuel is used throughout the course of the day.

• Mechanism •

The most important step in generating energy from glucose is glycolysis, which yields two molecules of pyruvic acid as its byproduct. It takes place in ten

subsequent chemical processes, resulting in a net gain of two ATP molecules from one glucose molecule. Only

around 43% of the available energy is used to create ATP, with heat making up the remaining 57% of the energy. The conversion of pyruvic acid to acetyl coenzyme A is the subsequent process. This reaction makes use of coenzyme A and results in the release of two molecules

of carbon dioxide and four hydrogen atoms. At this point, no ATP is produced, but the four hydrogen atoms that were released take part in oxidative phosphorylation, which leads to the release of six ATP molecules later. In the Krebs's cycle, also known as the tricarboxylic acid cycle, which takes place in the cytoplasm of the mitochondrion, acetyl coenzyme A is broken down, releasing energy in the form of ATP.

CHAPTER 4

•Glucose spike.

Although the term "glucose surge" isn't widely used, the experience it describes is probably:

A short boost in blood sugar is known as a glucose spike, and it is both normal and natural for people to experience one. A glucose spike is that momentary surge of energy that occurs in humans after eating candy, cookies, or other sweet foods, especially in children.

Rapid increases in blood sugar, however, might be hazardous for someone who has diabetes. Glucose spikes can cause the following symptoms in a diabetic person:

• Continual urination

Due to these consequences, it's critical for persons with diabetes to comprehend what triggers a glucose increase and how to minimize its effects.

Despite its unfavorable reputation, sugar is actually a crucial component of the human diet.

Although sugars occur in a wide variety of sizes and forms, most of them are converted into glucose during digestion.

When we consume, sugars from our food are transformed into glucose, which is then injected into the bloodstream, our body can use glucose to fuel all of its

essential processes. It is then transported throughout the body.

• As sugar is consumed and stored by cells, the amount of sugar in the blood gradually declines. However, people with diabetes struggle to control this process and may

experience very high glucose increases as a result (hyperglycemia).

Why does blood sugar spike?

Glucose spikes can happen for a variety of reasons, but the most frequent ones are forgetting to take an insulin shot, not exercising, and eating a lot of sugar.

It's important to note that other foods can also cause glucose levels to rise. The following foods frequently induce significant glucose spikes:

- Carbohydrates: These are foods that are starchy and high in complex sugars, such as bread, pasta, and potatoes.

- Fruits: Despite the fact that fruits provide vital vitamins, they also contain substantial amounts of sugar (often one called fructose)

- Alcohol: A few varieties of beers, wines, champagnes, and cocktails contain sugar and carbs.

- Since everyone reacts to foods differently, it's crucial to speak with a healthcare professional about the things you should be focusing on.

- Guidelines for Avoiding Blood Sugar Spikes.

Sharp increases in blood sugar are known as blood sugar spikes. They can be brought on by a number of things, but they frequently arise when you eat too many simple carbohydrates.

Blood sugar spikes are frequently caused by consuming excessive amounts of carbohydrates-containing food.

When you consume a meal that contains carbohydrates, your body converts the carbohydrates into glucose, a simple sugar. A signal is then sent to your pancreas telling it to release the hormone insulin as soon as the level of glucose in your blood starts to climb.

Blood Sugar Spike Symptoms.

• The more symptoms you are likely to have and the more harm your body is experiencing, the longer your blood sugar levels remain excessive. While hyperglycemia (high blood sugar) has some recognizable symptoms, they might differ from person to person.

• Minimizing any harm to your health and maintaining control of your diabetes can be accomplished by learning to detect your specific signs of high blood sugar early on.

High blood sugar is frequently accompanied by symptoms like frequent urination, increased thirst, constant hunger, blurry vision, fatigue, and headaches.

• Tingling or numbness in your hands or feet

• If any of these symptoms apply to you, have your blood sugar levels checked. It might be as easy as a small finger poke, yet it can help you regulate your blood sugar levels in a big way.

Visit a doctor as soon as you can if you do not have diabetes but are exhibiting any of these symptoms so that your blood sugar levels can be checked. Your life can be saved if diabetes and excessive blood sugar are detected early.

• The function of insulin is to function as a key to open the doors of various cells in your body. As a result, glucose can leave the bloodstream and enter the cells,

where it can either be used immediately for energy or stored for later. Without insulin, glucose builds up in the blood, leading to excessively high blood glucose (or blood sugar) levels. Serious health issues may result from this.

• In diabetes, insulin may occasionally be insufficient or malfunction. Due to this, it's crucial for diabetics to periodically check their blood sugar levels to ensure they are within a safe range.

How long do blood sugar peaks typically last?

• Blood sugar increases can last anywhere from a few minutes to several hours, depending on the individual and even the meal. Depending on what you ate, blood sugar increases typically start one to two hours after you start eating and can persist anywhere from a few minutes to several hours.

Nobody's plan, though, will work for everyone. The best course of action is for each person to develop their own meal plan with the assistance of a physician or nutritionist.

Chapter 5

The Glucogenic Diet

A diet can be accurately monitored by measuring portions.

Diabetes sufferers can benefit from a balanced, healthful diet that aids in controlling blood sugar levels.

This sort of diet development entails:

• Balancing carbohydrates, proteins, and lipids to achieve nutritional objectives

• Accurate portion measurement

• Forward planning

In light of this, the actions listed below could assist someone in creating a nutritious 7-day food plan:

1. Take note of the daily caloric and carbohydrate goals.

2. Calculate the number of servings of carbs and other meal ingredients necessary to reach those goals.

3. Distribute those servings throughout the meals and snacks of the day.

4. Review the rankings of favored and well-known foods and make an effort to include them in meals while taking into account the information above.

5. To fill out a daily plan, use exchange lists and other sources. Exchange lists categorize foods based on how many carbohydrates they have, making it easier to switch between different food types. Additionally, they could divide foods into subcategories and group those with comparable protein and fat contents.

6. Arrange your meals to make the most of your ingredients. For example, serve roast chicken one day and chicken soup the next.

7. Carry out this step again for every day of the week.

8. To determine whether the plan is having the desired effects, regularly check your weight and daily blood sugar levels

Considering meal preparation: the management of diabetes may be aided by meal planning. People with diabetes must balance their carbohydrate intake with their exercise levels, as well as their use of insulin and other medications.

- eating sufficient fiber to assist with dependable source blood sugar readings

- limiting foods with added sugars and highly processed carbs

- being aware of how dietary decisions can impact diabetes complications like high blood pressure

- maintaining a healthy weight

- paying attention to individualized treatment programs and advice from a physician or dietician

When making a diabetes meal plan, incorporating the various strategies listed below may be helpful.

glucose index

Foods are ranked on the glycemic index (GI) based on how rapidly their blood sugar levels are raised.

Blood sugar levels are quickly raised by foods with high GI ratings. Sugars and other carbs with a high level of processing are among these foods. Low-scoring foods either have no or few carbohydrates or have fiber, which takes longer for the body to absorb than processed carbohydrates.

Here are some examples of foods high in carbohydrates along with their GI ratings:

• Low GI (55 or less on the GI scale): Whole oats, most fruits, 100% stone-ground whole wheat bread, sweet potatoes with the skin, and whole grains.

Quick oats, brown rice, and whole wheat pita bread have a medium GI (56-69).

• High GI (70 and above) foods include melon, white bread, russet potatoes, candy, and white rice.

diet of 1,200 calories

The following meals and snacks make up the 1,200-calorie diet:

Monday

Breakfast consists of one orange, one poached egg, and half of a small avocado spread over Ezekiel toast. 39 carbohydrates in total.

Mexican bowl for *lunch*: two-thirds of a cup of low-sodium canned pinto beans, one cup of spinach that has been chopped, one ounce of cheese, one tablespoon of salsa, and four diced bell peppers. 30 carbohydrates in total.

20 1-gram baby carrots and 2 tablespoons of hummus for a snack. 21 carbohydrates in total.

Dinner will consist of one cup of cooked lentil penne pasta, two ounces of lean ground turkey, and one and a half cups of vegetarian tomato sauce with garlic, mushrooms, greens, zucchini, and eggplant. 35 carbohydrates in total.

125 grams of carbs total for the day.

Tuesday

Breakfast: 1/4 cup cooked oatmeal, 1/4 cup blueberries, 1/4-ounce almonds, and 1/4 tsp chia seeds. 34 carbohydrates in total.

Lunch: Salad ingredients: 12 cup chickpeas, 2 cups fresh spinach, 2 oz. grilled chicken breast, 12 small avocado, 14 cup shredded carrots, and 2 tbsp. dressing. 52 total carbohydrates.

Snack: 1/3 cup of 2% cottage cheese with 1 tiny peach sliced in it. 16 total carbohydrates.

Mediterranean couscous for dinner: two-thirds of a cup cooked whole wheat couscous, one tablespoon fresh basil, half a cup sautéed eggplant, five chopped jumbo olives, four sundried tomatoes, and half a cup diced cucumber. 38 carbohydrates in total.

140 carbohydrates altogether for the day.

Wednesday

Breakfast: a two-egg veggie omelet with spinach, mushrooms, bell pepper, avocado, and a third cup of blueberries. 34 carbohydrates in total.

Lunch: Sandwich: two regular slices of 100% whole wheat bread, one tablespoon of plain, nonfat Greek yogurt, one tablespoon of mustard, two ounces of canned tuna in water combined with one-quarter cup of shredded carrots, one-third of a tablespoon of dill relish, one cup of sliced tomato, and a half of a medium apple. 40 carbohydrates in total.

1 cup of unsweetened kefir as a snack. 12. Carbs overall.

Dinner will consist of 1 tsp. butter, 1/2 cup cooked asparagus, 2 oz. of pork tenderloin, and 1/2 cup fresh pineapple. 34 carbohydrates in total.

120 grams of carbs total for the day.

Thursday

breakfast will consist of two slices of toasted sweet potato topped with spinach, 1 teaspoon of flaxseed, and 1 oz of goat cheese. 44 carbohydrates in total.

Lunch: 1 cup of raw cauliflower, 2 ounces of roast chicken, 1 tablespoon of low-fat French dressing, and 1 cup of fresh strawberries. 23 carbohydrates in total.

Snack: Half a tiny banana and 1 cup plain, low-fat Greek yogurt. 15. Carbs overall.

Dinner will consist of two-thirds of a cup of quinoa, 8 oz. of silken tofu, 1 cup of cooked boc choy, 1 cup of steamed broccoli, 2 teaspoons of olive oil, and one kiwi. 44 carbohydrates in total.

Days' worth of carbohydrates: 126

FRIDAY

Breakfast should consist of a third cup of Grape-Nuts or another high-fiber cereal, half a cup of blueberries, and a cup of unsweetened almond milk. 41 total carbohydrates.

Lunch:

Salad: One boiled diced egg, two cups of spinach, one ounce of cheddar cheese, one-quarter cup of grapes, one

teaspoon of pumpkin seeds, and two ounces of roasted chickpeas make up this dish. 47 carbohydrates in total.

1 cup celery and 1 tablespoon peanut butter for a snack. six. Carbs overall

Dinner will consist of 1.5 cups of steamed asparagus, a medium baked potato, and a 2 oz. salmon filet. 39 carbohydrates in total.

133 total carbohydrates for the day.

Saturday

Breakfast: A cup of low-fat Greek yogurt with 1 cup strawberries, 1 cup mashed banana, and 1 tablespoon chia seeds. 32 carbohydrates in total.

Lunch: Two corn tortillas, one-third cup cooked black beans, one-ounce low-fat cheese, two tablespoons of avocado, one cup of coleslaw, and salsa as dressing. 70 grams in total.

Snack: 10 baby carrots, 1 cherry tomato, and 2 tablespoons hummus. 14 total carbohydrates.

Dinner will consist of a half-medium baked potato with the skin, 2 ounces of broiled steak, 1 teaspoon of butter, 1.5 cups of steamed broccoli, 1 teaspoon of nutritional yeast, and 3/4 cup of whole strawberries. 41 total carbohydrates.

157 total carbohydrates for the day.

SUNDAY

Breakfast: oats with chocolate and peanuts: One cup of cooked oatmeal, one scoop of chocolate soy or whey protein, one tablespoon of peanut butter, and one tablespoon of chia seeds. 21 total carbohydrates

Lunch: One small whole wheat pita pocket, half a cup of cooked lentils, half a cup of leafy greens, and three tablespoons of salad dressing. 30 carbohydrates in total.

Snack: 1 oz. of pumpkin seeds and 1 medium apple. 26 total carbohydrates.

3 ounces of boiled shrimp, 1 cup of green peas, 1 teaspoon of butter, 1/2 cup of beets, 1 cup of sautéed Swiss chard, and 1 teaspoon balsamic vinegar make up the dinner menu. 39 carbohydrates in total.

16 pistachios and 1 cup jicama for a snack. 15. Carbs overall.

131 total carbohydrates for the day.

limits on fruits

Fruit is quite nutrient-dense and may typically be included in a diabetes patient's balanced diet. The carbohydrate content of fruits should be taken into account, though, and diets should be modified as necessary. The American Diabetes Association recommends choosing fresh, tinned, or frozen fruits. Wherever possible, they ought to search for ones that are devoid of added sugars.

Although dried fruit and 100% fruit juice are both acceptable treats in moderation, whole fruits may be more filling.

A higher glycemic index may also be associated with some fruits, like as

• dates; ripe bananas; ripe pineapples; various dried fruits

• watermelon

Although one can use these in a diabetic diet plan, Precautions

A diabetes meal plan can make healthy eating more exciting by providing some fresh ideas to the diet while also assisting a person in keeping track of the calories and carbs they ingest. However, some people, including as those who are very physically active, those who are pregnant, breast- or chest-feeding, and those who have

specific medical issues, may not get enough calories from these meal plans.

A low-calorie diet can also be restricting and can make it harder to get the nutrients you need. Consequently, meticulous planning is crucial.

The following plans, which are based on estimations by the United States Department of Agriculture, include the number of carbohydrates for each meal and each day. They include three meals and snacks each day, all of which contain no more than three portions of nutritious, high-fiber carbs.

If a person is unsure about whether the numbers below are right for them, they should speak with a doctor or nutritionist. They can adjust as necessary by changing food proportions or adding supplements.

CONCLUSION

What does this all imply? It means that while fasting and post-meal glucose levels have defined "normal" ranges, these ranges do not clearly indicate what glucose trends should be over the course of a 24-hour period. Additionally, they don't state which ranges are ideal for the best health Because of repeated glucose peaks and valleys or excessive fasting glucose, even those with "normal" glucose levels may be at higher risk of health issues than they think. Your ideal glucose ranges are determined by a variety of personal circumstances, and they should be discussed with your healthcare professional. According to the studies, it's crucial to keep your blood sugar levels within the usual range and to avoid having too many spikes or dips. A customized diet

and lifestyle program that supports metabolic health should also achieve the following three objectives:

1. Reduce post-meal spikes in blood sugar

2. Maintain steady blood sugar levels and limit fluctuations in blood sugar throughout the day.

3. Strive to maintain fasting glucose levels at or below the "normal" range.

Iteratively identifying the diet and lifestyle choices that will help you reach these objectives is necessary; no one-size-fits-all approach is effective for everyone in maintaining blood glucose levels in the ideal range. By acting as a constant feedback mechanism, closing the loop between particular activities and the body's response, and paving the road for better present and future health, continuous glucose monitoring can assist you in establishing your ideal food and lifestyle choices.